The Basic Needs of a Woman

"...a thoughtful account of how to create conscious and meaningful births for mothers and their babies, and will encourage more compassionate care. Every woman should read it before going into labour, and then they should share their copy with all the maternity staff and vice versa. "

Robyn Sheldon - author of The Mama Bamba Way

"A jewel, a very precious one. Perfection. All men and women should read it and absorb it."

Liliana Lammers - doula and Paramana doula course facilitator

"Ruth Ehrhardt, you've combined the most wisdom regarding birth in such a short powerful read. I wish I had something like that before my births! I only read it after having 5 babies yet I learned things about the birth process because of your simple powerfully informed presentation that had escaped me in all my other reading!"

Becky Hastings, mother of five

"Being involved with the movement of natural and home birth in Brazil, I found your booklet one of the most useful pieces I have read about a woman in labour."

Vanessa Schultz, mother of three

The Basic Needs of a Woman in Labour

Ruth Ehrhardt

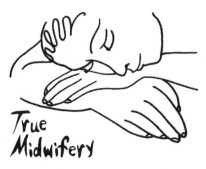

True
Midwifery

True Midwifery

Self published by Ruth Ehrhardt of True Midwifery

P O Box 44070, Scarborough, 7975, Western Cape, South Africa

www.truemidwifery.com

First published in South Africa in 2011

Book cover design by Ruth Ehrhardt and danielacc
Cover illustration by the travelerscat

Printed in South Africa

A catalogue record of this book is available from the National Library of South Africa

ISBN: 978-0-620-66028-0

When a woman births, not only is a baby being born but so is a mother.
How we treat her will affect how she feels about herself as a mother
and as a parent.
Be gentle. Be kind. Listen.

To every mother out there, may your birth be beautiful.

Foreword

There are two important published documents about birth physiology and the basic needs of labouring women. The first one is an enormous book written thousands of years ago. In the very first pages of this bestseller, there are some lines suggesting an association between the consumption of the fruit of the tree of knowledge (translate knowing too much or having developed a powerful neocortex) and the difficulties of human birth. At the end of this book, we can read about the birth of a legendary man whose mission was to promote love. His mother found a strategy to overcome the human handicap: with humility she gave birth among non-human mammals, in a stable.

The second document is the opposite of the first one in terms of size. It is a booklet by Ruth Ehrhardt. To bring together what is important in such a small number of pages is a feat. I hope that, on the five continents, all pregnant women, midwives, doulas, doctors, etc. will take the time to assimilate the contents of this chef d'oeuvre: it will be a turning point in the history of childbirth and therefore in the history of mankind.

- **Michel Odent**

Introduction

This booklet is inspired by the work of Dr. Michel Odent.

Dr. Odent started his medical career as a surgeon and became involved in birth when he was put in charge of a hospital in Pithiviers, outside Paris. He soon realised that hospitals were not conducive to a woman in labour. They were too bright, sterile and uncomfortable and lacked privacy. He was the first person to introduce low beds (easier for a labouring woman to climb in and out of), dim lighting, beautiful home-like rooms, and eventually water as a form of pain relief, in a hospital setting.

The hospital in Pithiviers was so successful that many people came specially to have their babies there. Dr. Odent was there from 1962 to 1985. He worked with six midwives and oversaw approximately 1000 births per year. The hospital's maternity section had excellent statistics with low rates of intervention.

He eventually moved to London and became a home birth midwife there. Again, he was able to make many interesting observations through his experience there.

Later he founded the Primal Health Research Centre (see www.primalhealthresearch.com).

For the last 12 years he has been working with a doula called Liliana Lammers. Together they run the Paramana Doula course in London.

Liliana is a quiet and unassuming woman who holds an incredible strength in doing very little at a birth. She is able to hold a space with her presence alone, a quiet strength. She must make a woman feel very safe in labour.

Through his many years (more than half a century) of attending births (around 15 000 births) in both hospitals and at home, Dr. Odent has come to the conclusion that a labouring woman needs not much more than to be left alone, simply to be attended to by a quiet, non-invasive and low profile midwife.

This little booklet is a summary of what I have learned from attending Michel Odent and Liliana Lammer's course in December 2010, by reading Michel's books, and from my own experience and work with pregnant and labouring women.

I hope it can be helpful to you.

Ruth Ehrhardt
Red Hill
Cape Town
South Africa
2011

When a Woman is Pregnant

When a woman is pregnant she is very sensitive. There is a baby growing inside her and her body is changing. Much of her strength and energy is being used to create the building blocks of a new person and she might feel tired and nauseous, and be more sensitive to food. She will often feel very strange and different.

Her emotions will also be effected by this new change in her body and in her life. For this reason she needs to feel that those around her care about her and about how she feels. She needs people around her who will listen to her, especially to listen to how she feels about her pregnancy and the coming birth and about having a new baby. Being there for a woman in pregnancy can mean listening to any problems she may be having in her life, or it could mean bringing her some good food, or washing the dishes for her. Her body is working very hard to grow a new baby for this world. She needs help from her friends, family and community if she is going to be able to be healthy and strong during this time.

A pregnant woman needs to eat good, healthy food, and she needs to rest when she is tired. A pregnant woman needs to have fun. She is growing a baby but this doesn't mean that she doesn't want to have fun! The more a pregnant woman enjoys herself, the more good feelings go to her baby. Babies can feel what their mothers feel. If a mother is sad or angry the baby feels it. If the mother is feeling happy and loved, the baby feels happy and loved too.

A pregnant woman can enjoy herself in many ways. She can sing or dance or read a book or watch a movie or be with friends. She can go for a walk on the beach. It is also enjoyable to be with other pregnant women and to be with women who have had babies and who have good stories to tell about their births and about being mothers.

It is important to realise that our words can have a very strong effect on a pregnant woman. While we do not have to paint a flowery picture of pregnancy, birth and parenthood, we can be aware that it is not productive to dwell on the difficulties (the nausea, the heartburn, the swollen ankles, the tiredness). We need to remember and tell her of the exhilaration of birth and its beauty.

We must remember that the smallest thing can make a pregnant woman anxious. Caregivers sometimes don't realise how much power their words have and how much their words can influence an expectant mother's feelings. Many women leave their antenatal appointments feeling very worried about their or their baby's health. That something is wrong with them and often they feel guilty. Caregivers should remember this before they tell a woman that they think that her baby may be too big, or that she has too much or too little amniotic fluid, or that her blood pressure is too high, or that there is sugar in her urine. Unless there is a real and present danger they should not worry a pregnant woman and her family unnecessarily.

Worry during pregnancy can be harmful and counterproductive.

When a Woman is in Labour

Going into labour is like falling asleep...

Labour is a different state of being, a state of being with a lot of similarities to sleep. For a start they are both states that cannot be forced. They just happen! Sometimes when we least expect it. We cannot decide or control the moment when we fall asleep. We can also not decide or control the moment when we "fall into labour." But we *can* make it difficult for both to happen easily and most effectively.

Labour is like sleep because we need the same conditions to "fall into labour" as we need to "fall asleep." We need to feel safe and warm and relaxed. We need to be in a place in which we feel comfortable, and we need to be free from pressure, anxiety or fear.

Oxytocin

When a woman is in labour she releases a hormone called oxytocin. Oxytocin is the hormone that makes the uterus contract during labour.

It is also the hormone of **love**.

Oxytocin is the hormone we release when we are enjoying a meal, or having a stimulating conversation. It is the hormone we release when we are making love and when we orgasm. It is the hormone that makes us feel in love, and it is the hormone that releases the milk when a mother is breastfeeding.

Isn't it amazing that it is the *love* hormone that brings the baby into the world?

In hospitals synthetic oxytocin is often given to women. It has different names like **Pitocin** or **Syntocinon**. Synthetic oxytocin is given to make the mother's uterus contract, which can help to birth the baby. But this synthetic oxytocin is not a love hormone. It is not like the oxytocin that is naturally secreted by the mother's body. Synthetic oxytocin is just a hormone that contracts the uterus and helps to push the baby out. It is important that we know more about the effects and function of natural oxytocin, because when a labouring woman is under the effect of synthetic oxytocin she may have a decreased ability to produce natural oxytocin.

How is synthetic oxytocin used?

Synthetic oxytocin is used to **induce** a labour (this means starting a labour artificially) or to **augment** a labour (this means to speed up a labour that has stopped or slowed down). Synthetic oxytocin is also used for **active management of the third stage of labour** when the placenta is delivered (an injection of synthetic oxytocin is given to the mother to help deliver the placenta quickly). It is also used to stop a mother bleeding if she has a **post partum haemorrhage** (when the mother's uterus doesn't contract after birth and she begins to bleed heavily).

Induction

These days it is very common for a woman to be induced to start her labour. She may be given many reasons for this: she may be over her due date, or her caregivers may be worried that her baby is getting too big, or that her baby is ill, or that she is ill.

Augmentation

When a woman is in labour, it is common for her labour to slow down or even to stop when she arrives in hospital. There could be many reasons for this sudden slowing down of the labour: the lights are too bright, she is given a vaginal examination, a stranger enters the room, she is feeling watched or self conscious, she is feeling rushed, cold or scared. Usually, if the labour doesn't start up again after a certain amount of time, synthetic oxytocin will be used to get the labour going again. This labour is now very different to the natural labour of the love hormone. This new labour is now governed by a synthetic oxytocin, which has the effect of contracting the uterus *without* the behavioural effects of the natural love hormone.

*The baby, when he
or she is ready to
be born,
will send a message
that tells the
mother's body that
it is ready.*

*The mother's body
can then begin
labour by slowly
releasing oxytocin,
the hormone of
love.*

*The mother and
baby work together
to bring the baby
into the world.*

How does oxytocin work?

Oxytocin is a shy hormone....

Oxytocin needs to feel comfortable before being released. Since it is the love hormone this makes sense. When we are feeling in love we feel safe. Love is not something that is easy to feel when we are in danger.

Oxytocin is a fussy hormone. Everything needs to be just right for this hormone to want to make an entrance. The more comfortable the environment and the more relaxed the labouring woman, the more her oxytocin will be able to flow.

A sense of security

The labouring woman needs to feel secure and safe. Mammals will find a secure place to give birth. A wonderful example is female elephants who will form a circle around the labouring mother elephant with their backs turned to her.

If a labouring mammal feels threatened her labour will stop until she is in a safe place again. Human beings are not that different physiologically. We also are mammals after all. While many women choose to give birth in hospitals because they feel it is their safest option, they may find that when they arrive at the hospital their bodies react in a way which tells us that they are not feeling safe in that environment. The bright lights, the talking, the signing of papers, the questions, having to interact with strangers, the ticking clock, the cold sterile rooms, the high beds, the lack of privacy, the foetal heart monitors... these can all contribute to a feeling of being unsafe. This may make it difficult for oxytocin, the shy hormone, to makes its appearance. One can then anticipate a longer and more difficult labour.

How do other mammals prepare for birth? They will find a quiet, dark place, far away from anyone, somewhere where they will feel safe and secure and know that they will be undisturbed.

A woman at the end of her pregnancy is much the same. We joke about the 'nesting instinct' when a woman at the end of her pregnancy frantically cleans her home in preparation for the birth. Some women cannot rest until the curtains are hung just right or the floors are scrubbed or all her affairs are put to rest. Doing this makes it possible for them to feel ready to have their baby

The thinking brain needs to switch off
One of the prime ingredients for shy oxytocin to take effect is that the thinking brain needs to switch off. We need to make sure that the labouring woman's thinking brain (called the **neo-cortex**) is not stimulated.

We stimulate the neo-cortex during labour by talking to the labouring woman about logical things, such as telling her how many centimetres dilated she is, or asking her to remember when her waters broke. We stimulate her neo-cortex with these observations and questions, and as a result we slow down her release of oxytocin.

A woman needs to be able to slowly fall into her labour (like falling asleep) and not be 'woken up' by the outside world. If she can be given the space to switch off her neo-cortex, oxytocin will be able to do its job.

No observers
Feeling observed also stimulates the neo-cortex, so it is important that the mother does not feel watched. Observers and unnecessary people make the mother feel observed. Cameras can also slow labour down because they can make a mother feel observed which will "wake her up."

Darkness
It is important that there are no bright lights around a labouring woman. Drawn curtains, candles and other dim lighting will help to suppress the thinking brain and aid in the stimulation of oxytocin.

Warmth
The labouring woman needs to be warm. A fire or a heater or warm water is helpful in relaxing her body and her neo-cortex. In fact, immersing herself in warm water at the right time (when she is in established active labour) can relax the mother so much that her cervix will dilate completely.

Oxytocin/adrenaline antagonism
Adrenaline prevents oxytocin from being released. Adrenaline is the hormone we produce when we are frightened, anxious, stressed or cold. It is known as the 'fight or fright' hormone. Adrenaline *suppresses* oxytocin. It can completely stop labour or make the labour longer and more painful.

Anyone who is present at a birth needs to very aware of his or her levels of adrenaline. This is because adrenaline is contagious, which means that if you are feeling anxious or scared or nervous, everyone else in the room will soon start feeling that way too. If you are at a birth and you are feeling tense or nervous or scared, try to calm yourself down. If you can't, it will serve the mother better if you leave the room until you are feeling better.

Have a look around and see how the other people in the room are behaving. If you can see that someone is feeling uncomfortable, you can gently let that person know that it is okay for him or her to take a break and perhaps leave the room, or go for a walk, or try to have a sleep. This must be done in a gentle and non-aggressive way because if you get angry or make someone else angry you will create more adrenaline.

Sometimes people are relieved to be told that they can take a break from the birth. A birth is a very intense experience, which can be very overwhelming.

The Basic Needs of a Woman in Labour Are:

- To feel safe
- To leave the thinking brain (the neo-cortex) switched off
- Silence
- Darkness or low lights
- Warmth
- Not feeling observed
- No adrenaline

A basic birth plan

(insert place)

Labour Partners

1. my husband / partner

2. my doula

For any questions throughout labour please don't ask me but my doula or my husband.

Monitoring baby and I:

• If there's a real need for a vaginal exam, please don't share with me the details of how dilated I am and the baby's position.

• Listen to the baby's heartbeat as little as possible, it could disturb my labour.

• If there's a need to listen to baby's heartbeat, please do so without asking permission, so I do not need to think to give you an answer.

• Please don't offer me pain relief. If I need some I'll ask for it myself.

2nd & 3rd stages of labour:

• Immediately after birth I'd like one hour uninterrupted skin-to-skin with my baby.

• Please do not clamp/cut the cord until 1 hour after the birth of my baby.

• I would like physiological third stage, as long as labour progresses normally.

After the birth:

• Vitamin K? (you decide) three choices: injected, oral or no Vitamin K for my baby.

The Birth Attendant

The perfect birth attendant is a silent, low profile midwife...

The ideal birth attendant should preferably be a mother herself, someone who has a positive attitude towards birth. She would have had positive birth experiences herself.

She is there to make the labouring mother feel safe. To provide a sense of security.

She views birth as normal and understands the environmental factors that need to be in place for oxytocin to flow.

She understands that talking and asking questions will stimulate the labouring mother's neo-cortex. Therefore she keeps talking to a minimum and will try to answer as many questions as possible on behalf of the labouring mother. This way the mother doesn't need to be 'woken up' from her labour.

The ideal birth attendant knows that bright lights stimulate the neo-cortex and so she makes sure that the lights are dimmed or off or that the curtains are drawn during the day.

The ideal birth attendant knows that the labouring mother needs to be warm in order to relax and for her oxytocin to release and flow. She makes sure that the room is sufficiently heated and knows that a warm shower or bath can work very well as a form of pain relief.

The ideal birth attendant knows that the labouring mother must feel uninhibited and should not feel that she is being observed. The birth attendant keeps her eyes averted. She also knows that cameras and video cameras can make a mother feel observed and can slow the labour down.

The ideal birth attendant keeps her own adrenaline levels low – she is very aware of herself and the effect that she has on the labouring mother and others.

The ideal birth attendant trusts that the birthing process will take its natural course and that the mother and baby are the main actors.

Above all the ideal birth attendant provides a **sense of security**. She protects the birthing environment and makes the mother feel safe.

The ideal birth attendant will bring a sense of security with her presence alone.

The Fetus Ejection Reflex

One cannot help an involuntary process, the point is not to disturb it...

If the labouring mother has had her basic needs met during the first stages of her labour, her body will prepare itself for something called the **Fetus Ejection Reflex.**

It is very important that the labouring mother has utmost privacy during this time, otherwise the fetus ejection reflex will not take place.

How does it occur?
When a fetus ejection reflex is about to take place, the mother will suddenly become fearful and will say things like: "I want to die!" or "Kill me!"

It would be a mistake at this point to try to soothe or placate the mother with reassuring words.

Soon after this there will be some very strong contractions. The labouring mother will suddenly be full of energy and she will want to be upright.

The baby will be expelled in a few strong contractions. The Fetus Ejection Reflex is different from what we know as the **second stage of labour,** which is when the mother has to actively push the baby out.

When a true fetus ejection reflex takes place, the likelihood of the mother tearing is very low and the placenta should only take a few minutes to separate.

A fetus ejection reflex **cannot** take place if the basic needs of a woman in labour have not been met.

After the Birth

Do not wake the mother!

When the baby is born he or she should be placed on the mother's bare skin and they should be left alone and **undisturbed** for at least an hour.

This means *no fiddling*!

No one should talk. **No one** should take photos.

All one needs to do is to make sure that the mother and baby are warm.

Once the baby is born, the mother will release a massive surge of oxytocin. This is the highest level of oxytocin she will ever experience in her life. The oxytocin will make her fall in love and bond with her baby. It will also help her placenta to release and her uterus to clamp down.

During the first hour after birth the baby will be adapting to the effect of gravity and the change in temperature. This is the perfect time for mother and baby to initiate breastfeeding all on their own.

Cord Cutting
There is no reason to rush to cut the umbilical cord after the birth. Try to leave the cord for at least an hour after the birth.

There is no harm in this.

The cord between the placenta and the baby contains two arteries and a vein. The arteries close within a few minutes but the vein remains open, so the baby can gain up to 40ml of precious blood.

Cord cutting is a ritual
For thousands of years, mankind has interfered with the first contact between mother and baby.

Over the centuries and in different cultures, mothers have not been allowed to touch their babies unless given permission by the midwife or father or a priest. Some cultures said that colostrum (the first 'milk' the mother produces for the first few days after giving birth which is highly nutritious and full of anti bodies) was poisonous and therefore the baby would have to be fed gruel or another animal's milk or milk from another woman. Some cultures cheer loudly as the baby is born, 'waking' the mother. Others need to clean or pass the baby over smoke before it is handled by the mother.

Our modern day ritual is to congratulate the mother, cut the cord hurriedly deliver the placenta, check for tears, take photos, weigh and measure the baby, invite others into the room to view the baby and to discuss the birth and baby with the mother.

It is a strange fact that one of the greatest discoveries of the 20th century is that **a baby needs its mother in the moments after birth**.

Now it seems that we need to discover that it needs its mother and *nobody else.*

The Future

Today the majority of women are giving birth without the use of their natural hormones.

Their labours are induced.

Or augmented.

Many are giving birth via caesarean.

Even if they give birth without intervention, that sacred first hour after birth will be disturbed.

We are changing the way women give birth.

We are making these changes without an understanding of the basic needs of a woman in labour.

We are making these changes without much knowledge of what effect this will have on the future.

A Story

A midwife sits in a dark room.

She has a shawl wrapped around her shoulders.

A candle flickers on the table.

She is knitting.

From another room, you hear the soft moan of a woman. The midwife continues knitting. The woman in the other room becomes silent again.

The midwife continues knitting. After a few minutes you hear the moan from the other room again and the midwife smiles to herself while she continues to knit.

Some time goes by and the midwife gets up and leaves the room. She goes to the kitchen. You hear her switch on the kettle.

The labouring woman continues to moan and groan - the pains seem to be intensifying.

The midwife comes back with a steaming cup of tea and a plate of biscuits. She dips her biscuits and sips her tea.

The labouring woman continues to moan softly in the next room.

The midwife is sitting on a rocking chair and now she rocks herself quietly while the woman in labour continues with her noises.

The midwife falls asleep.

The midwife sleeps for a while, while the mother's noises intensify.

The mother begins to shriek. She feels that the pain is too much. She is afraid that she is going to die.

The midwife opens her eyes and quietly listens. She slowly gets up (her bones creak a little) and she shuffles out of the room towards the sounds of the labouring woman.

Quietly, like a cat, the midwife slips into the room where the mother is.

The mother is grunting and screaming and the baby is born.

The baby is crying.

The midwife comes out of the room.

The mother is cooing to her baby.

The midwife shuffles back to her chair, sits down, smiles softly to herself and continues to knit.

About the Author

Ruth Ehrhardt is a Certified Professional Midwife and a doula.

Originally born in Switzerland, Ruth Ehrhardt moved to South Africa with her South African born mother and younger sister when she was eight years old and has lived there ever since. Ruth's mother Carol bought a protea flower farm an hour outside of Ceres (a small town, approximately 2 1/2 hours from Cape Town) and accidentally 'fell' into catching the babies of the local farm labourers who called for her because she had 'healing hands.' Carol was the midwife for Ruth's first birth.

The mother of four home birthed children, Ruth first trained as a WOMBS doula with Irene Bourquin in South Africa and later attended the Paramana doula course with Dr Michel Odent and Lilliana Lammers in London. She has also studied Advanced Midwifery with Ina May Gaskin, Pamela Hunt and the Farm Midwives.

With colleague Lana Petersen, she started Home Birth South Africa (www.homebirth.org.za), a web data base for those seeking information and advice on home birth in South Africa. Together, they also run the Cape Town Home Birth Gatherings, a quarterly gathering for those seeking information and support on home birth.

She is currently working with Marianne Littlejohn of Birthrite Midwifery and is one of the organisors of The Cape Town Midwifery and Birth Conference (www.midwiferyandbirthconference.co.za) - a conference organised to encourage sharing and collaboration between birthing professionals and the women they serve. This conference was a first of its kind in South Africa and was met with resounding success.

She is also trained as a Helping Babies Breathe Facilitator and master trainer.

She is an advocate for women's, mothers' and babies' rights and is involved in various projects to further education and support in these areas.

She regularly writes on her personal website and blog www.truemidwifery.com.

Note from Author

This book has been very well received by most who have read it. The idea was to make a summary of something so simple and yet so overlooked. Something which can make all the difference at a birth, to the mother, to her baby and to the future of mankind.

It is my mission to spread this little yet powerful message as far and as wide as possible and I have started by writing this little book which is easy to read and understand and inexpensive to reproduce.

I would like to translate this work into as many as languages as possible - if you would like to help with this please let me know.

Also, I am seeking honest reviews for the book on Amazon and whilst I would appreciate it if you find the time, after reading the book, to leave a review, you are by no means obliged to do so. Feel free to post your thoughts directly to Amazon, I would appreciate your thoughts, both positive and negative.

Thank you,

Ruth Ehrhardt
Suurbraak/X!airu
South Africa
2013

For more information see Michel Odent's websites

www.wombecology.com

www.primalhealthresearch.com

You can contact Ruth Ehrhardt at

ruth@homebirth.org.za

Ruth's personal website is:

www.truemidwifery.com

Printed in Great Britain
by Amazon

43896300R00020